Enjoy Eating Less

Letters to a Grandchild

Warning

If the language used seems harsh or unfashionable, clarity demands robust, accurate use of words. For example 'obese', often used as a term of abuse, occurs here in its precise clinical definition: BMI (body mass index) over 30.

'Normal' has recently become taboo in educational or psychiatric contexts; the advice is to replace it by 'average'. As this is not a true equivalent, 'normal' occurs here with its traditional connotations. Tolerance of demonizing many words in current usage leads to general impoverishment of our language.

ISBN #: 978-1-4457-3192-6

Content ID: 8519826

This 2010 edition is dedicated to Madeline, who has accepted with equanimity the implied slur in the title, that her culinary accomplishment, over the 61 years of our marriage, has been enjoyed more by eating less of it

Contents

Preface

When so much daunting material has been written about weight loss, a preface must explain and excuse yet another addition to what is available on obesity in books, magazines, newspaper articles, on TV, and now on the Internet. This booklet is needed because plans on offer to achieve weight loss lack common sense, are impractical, cranky or patronizing, and do not work long term. The April '03 study of the four most popular (and profitable) dietary schemes used in the UK (see Letter 19) showed none of them helped 94% of the volunteers taking part, confirmed by a later survey in June '06. If this is the best the four most popular schemes can offer, the need for a different approach is imperative.

Obesity is a moral problem, not a medical one. Those affected must be responsible for solving their weight problem. The pretence that doctors can cure this moral problem has made it worse; it is also foolish because the failure was predictable. Attempts to coerce patients to diet or alter their eating habits don't work. The 'epidemic' of obesity is said to be 'out of control' because no funds are available to train the large number of obesity experts needed to solve the problem.

Nevertheless doctors will persevere, adding to the incidence of iatrogenic disease. For those unfamiliar with this term, it is defined as 'caused by medically prescribed treatment'. With the powerful drugs now available for almost every disease, increase of iatrogenic disease is inevitable. The complications of obesity: cardiovascular, orthopaedic, diabetic and many others, require medical treatment involving yet more iatrogenic disease.

To those doctors who believe many of the overweight or obese are guilty of gluttony, the victims could validly reply that those doctors are guilty of pride. Aggravating the situation, the bureaucrats, a third party in an unholy trinity, are eager to provide clinics for the participants. From these they will superintend the pretended treatment. Apologizing is much in vogue for mistakes in the distant past. Should doctors apologize for the increase of iatrogenic disease as it is caused by medically prescribed treatment, or will the Department of Health as the overriding authority accept the blame?

When a grandchild in her last year at school asked for help, a few pages of advice, based on the system I had used a few years previously, though gratefully received, were not as successful as she and I had hoped. It lacked sustainability. To succeed with a new way of eating requires more consistent help than a single page of advice.

To relieve pressure on worn-out knees, I had needed to shed 3st 2lb (20 kg). The method I had offered to patients worked; weight lost and not regained. It was more difficult than expected and I was reminded of Dr James Le Fanu's observation that only when a doctor experiences treatment or illness, does he realize the difficulties his patients have borne without complaint when similarly afflicted. The practical difficulties were apparent, but not until I needed to describe the details, did I fully realize how those difficulties should be confronted.

Following a suggestion from Dr Le Fanu, the advice was converted into weekly letters to the grandchild. They proved successful, not only for her but also for many others who learnt about them from his column in *The Daily Telegraph* 2001. This format was said to be unacceptable for commercial publication, so the 'letters' were changed to mini-chapters for the 2004 edition.

Six years later the material needs updating after advice from colleagues, friends and especially from readers of the 3500 booklets sent out. Readers have welcomed the approach to slimming that advocates a retreat from 'dieting'. I am grateful for their useful suggestions that are included in this revision (March 2010). They endorse the principle they know best how to decide what to eat. They find reliance on that principle preferable to conflicting advice from 'experts' who bombard us with unwanted edicts. For further information on why current advice from the Department of Health is not appropriate see the Appendix.

Simpler, more sensible options are urgently needed, which governments, professions and ordinary individuals with a sense of responsibility should support now. The original format of 'Letters to a Grandchild' is reinstated to emphasize the importance of individual advice. This contrasts with DoH information targeted at the amorphous collection of 'average' citizens. The DoH advice is not helpful because it does not address the many and varied problems of the suffering obese. Their 'advice' comes from deskbound authority, with no practical experience of dealing with individual patients (clients) and is aimed at the 'average'. Contrast this with the targeted individual advice offered by practising GPs like Dr James Le Fanu to which his readers warm.

Acknowledgments

Dr James le Fanu suggested the format of Letters to a Grandchild. It made the advice cogent, acceptable and successful. His support and commendation of succeeding versions encouraged me to persevere.

Dr Stefan Waydenfeld (whom I knew through Dr Le Fanu's recommendation of his excellent book *The Ice Road*) advised his patients that losing weight involved changing of eating habits for the rest of their lives; this agrees with the views expressed here. I am grateful for his percipient, constructive and valued comments.

John Ryan, my contemporary, has been a friend for over 70 years. His Captain Pugwash enlivens the front cover, providing light relief. Sadly he died in 2009.

Richard Jeffrey-Gray of Hoxa has been a tower of strength producing 3 editions of this booklet – endlessly patient and a reliable source of excellent practical advice.

I thank many colleagues for checking the accuracy of the advice, and to readers and friends who have suggested alterations.

John Mountford, author of *An Insight into English Spelling,* has proof read the text, adding clarity; remaining weaknesses show where his advice has been ignored.

I am grateful to **Professor Stanley Feldman, Professor Vincent Marks** and the 16 other contributors to the essays: "*Unpicking the Myths we're told about Food and Health*" – the subtitle of *Panic Nation* published July 2005. Many subjects considered in *Panic Nation* provide scientific justification for assertions made on common sense grounds in *Enjoy Eating Less*. It is a relief to find such a raft of expert opinion to sustain those assumptions. Professor Stanley Feldman has encouraged me to persevere in challenging some of the current Department of Health policies on food and health matters.

James (my nephew) and **Jenny Mountford** keep me up-to-date with current medical developments. They introduced me to Dr Ben Goldacre's *Bad Science.* They qualified with him and also introduced *Enjoy Eating Less* to medical circles in the USA.

Professor Gareth Greenslade gave a memorable lecture on Obesity to the Bristol Medchi Society and has provided practical advice about getting this latest revised version published.

Last but not least I am grateful to **Helen**, recipient of the original letters, whose patient imperturbability, willing co-operation and sensible questions encouraged me to write more than I originally planned.

Introduction

*There is nothing original in advocating eating less to produce weight loss. The unwelcome negative message is repeated or implied by every purveyor of schemes to combat obesity. It is unusual to combine it with the positive, liberating, revolutionary advice to enjoy eating what **you** like, not what someone else tells you.*

Individual accounts of eating less, as for example by Lord Lawson, usually describe a series of menus. They may be interesting as anecdotal evidence of success for the person describing them, they sell well but they are of little practical use for most of us, for whom the individual menus, often exotic, will be quite unsuitable. It is not derogatory to say this; Nigel Lawson's admirable example should be followed, but we must also copy him in devising and deciding our own menus and speed of weight loss.

The emphasis here is not only on the general application of *non-dietary eating less*, but how much more effective it is when we choose our own menus. It will work for any rational person prepared to confront the difficulties involved. The great boon is the shifting of responsibility from the advice-giver to the advice taker. To prevent the most common failure – weight regained – we must never go back to eating more than we need. Changing eating habits for the rest of your life is obligatory, and is a vital part of the plan. Not dieting – but a realistic acknowledgment that *eating more than each of us needs is the immediate cause of obesity.* Remote or subsidiary causes – viruses, genetic, addiction to hamburgers – are irrelevant, only of academic interest. Let us leave these considerations to academics because the *sole* effective treatment is rigorous control of food intake.

This approach has been criticized as over-simplified; I take this as a compliment. Causes of obesity are diagnosed in contradictory and mutually incompatible ways (see Letter 9);

clarification is needed. A small but important part of a GP's role has always been to clarify consultants' expert opinions to patients. When offered multiple causes of obesity, it is sensible to consider the most likely. To diagnose most overweight and obese people as having a metabolic disorder (see Dr Atkins New Diet, Letter 19) is as unreasonable as to believe that they are all food addicts (Letter 20) or suffer from lack of self-esteem – a psychiatric view.

The link between affluence and increased food consumption is obvious; the common sense conclusion: eating more than we need is the prime cause of obesity. The simple cure, *eating less*, is equally obvious. Though simple it works. Such advice is ignored by the food industry and its advertising accomplices who encourage us to eat more than we need. Nor do the multi-million pounds slimming industry welcome it, nor those who provide keep-fit gym-exercise centres and rely on regular contributions from the overweight. The latter will save money by eating less and stop paying those eager to counsel and control them.

The primary need for this advice is to accept responsibility so it is not suitable for the irresponsible, or for those who are, for whatever reason, irrational. Excluding these means that some will not be helped. However with over 50% of us overweight or obese, many want a rational way to lose weight with good prospects of success. None of the fashionable methods currently recommended by the DoH or the slimming industry are suitable or likely to succeed. This plan might not help all of the depressed or melancholic though it can help some. Those needing or receiving psychiatric care are well catered for by many special programmes to combat obesity.

For those with common sense, who are averse to being counselled or to employing a personal trainer or guru, who are rational, self-reliant, individualistic, optimistic, open to new ideas but resistant to the latest fashion, the only essential advice is that **it is not *what* we eat that matters, but *how much.***

24 Letters to a Grandchild

A set of weekly letters to a grandchild is at the heart of *Enjoy Eating Less*. They describe a do it yourself common sense guide to the logic of non-diet slimming. This is a prescription to be followed not medicine to be swallowed. Whether the letters should be read weekly or at one go is up to the individual. Unlike most prescriptions the risk of overdosing is minimal.

The prescription to be 'authentic' in line with cigarette packets and now wine bottles, should have a Government Warning, listing known side effects with instructions to report any new ones.

The official reaction to common sense is dismissive – how can anyone be so frivolous about the grave problem of obesity by having a comic cartoon on the cover and the word *Enjoy* as the title's first word? Encouraging the populace to use common sense, or take an initiative contradicting the official view must be challenged.

The official response is predictable: *This advice trivializes a serious problem. It has not been peer-reviewed. Science is already decided. Obesity experts have been considering the problem for many years. They need more funds to deliver a report pointing the way forward.*

Side effects, listed in enormous numbers, more varied than can be imagined, are printed in tiny type, illegible without a magnifying glass, should apply to these letters. Readers who recognise side effects should decide to whom they should be reported

Letter 1: The Plan

Dear H

The Plan is absurdly simple. There are three basic principles:

1) **Choice**: Eat what **you** like, not what someone tells you, but **much less** of it

2) **Moderation:** Avoid extremes

3) **Common sense:** Take responsibility yourself

   There is no list of forbidden foods, no calorie counting or weighing what you eat.

Note the lack of detail and no menus. The vital ingredient is that it is tailored to the individual, who must make all the decisions. No one else has the right to tell us what we should eat and what we should avoid. Accepting responsibility is a recipe for success. Surrendering independence to those unqualified to advise is not.

*Stage 1: To lose weight, food intake must be restricted to **less than the body needs,** forcing the body to burn up surplus fat – difficult but not impossible. Use this time to practice the important learning experience of changing eating habits, essential to prevent the lost weight being regained.*

Stage 2: A more relaxed time, gradually increase your intake, but stop the weight returning by abandoning your old eating habits.

Obesity was described in the *British Medical Journal* (Oct 2002) as an untreatable epidemic, re-emphasized in the *BMJ* (Sep & Dec 2006) as out of control – a pessimistic counsel of despair because an epidemiological approach is unworkable. While suitable for a cholera outbreak – a water-borne infection has to be cured by those in charge of the water supply – it cannot solve a problem affecting only part of the population. Draconian imposition of dietary changes, banning of so-called 'junk food' cannot be imposed on the unaffected (nearly half the population). Even applying dietary restrictions only to the overweight would be ineffective because each of us reacts differently. Some might respond others would not. The sensible answer is to persuade the overweight and obese to be responsible for their problem.

This Plan will cure an individual who is obese or overweight. If everyone took this advice, the 'epidemic' would be treatable; because many will not responsible individuals need not despair. When enough follow this route, their example should encourage others. The possibility of the obesity problem being solved will be glimpsed. It is absurd to believe obesity per se is untreatable. Help is at hand for the individual, Suitably modified for each of us, this Plan works. Just follow the general principles. Why will it, when other plans don't? Because most of us will not obey imposed rules. Those who lose weight, quickly regain it.

The first principle is clear, simple, self-explanatory: **"Eat what you like but much less of it"**. It could be criticised as imprecise, vague, even woolly, but the implied change in eating habits is the heart of the matter. It allows for infinite variation, to suit each; our needs vary widely. The lack of precision is its virtue. It has to be tailored to suit our varied responses.

The Department of Health (supported by TV nutritionists) tells us to avoid *'junk food'* and plans to ban it. *'Junk food'* – a contradiction of terms – comes high in any list of oxymorons. An item is either nutritious, in which case it is a food, or it has no nutritional value, and can be classed as junk. It cannot be both. How legislation will define junk food remains to be seen, but food suppliers will resist their product being so classified. More appropriate for them to carry a warning label: *"This is so highly nutritious (packed with calories) it should be taken with care – share it with a friend."*

Letter 2: Target Weight: Choose your own, using the Table

Dear H

Body Mass Index: The weight in kilograms divided by the square of the height in metres, a calculation impossible without using a slide rule (obsolete) or calculator. Few people in the UK know their weight in kilograms, even fewer their height in metres; so, ignoring inevitable criticism from those who disapprove the use of inches, stones or pounds, the same ratio can be calculated with imperial units: the **BMI is the weight in pounds multiplied by 703, divided by the square of the height in inches**. *While still a less than friendly calculation, it does use familiar units and it is the BMI ratio in universal use. To save the tedium of calculating your BMI (or that of your friends), and of what you would like it to be, the table shows the weight in stones and pounds for different heights in feet and inches for 5 key BMI figures. It shows, for your height, what experts believe it should be; less helpfully it tells you how tall you should be for your present weight. Decide the weight you would like to be yourself.*

How can you diagnose being overweight? Look at yourself nude in a full-length mirror; using two mirrors provides a more realistic if disturbing image. Before BMI, "normal" weight was estimated from weight and height charts used by insurance companies to load premiums for those who were outside chosen limits with separate charts for men and women. As life expectancy differs it was prudent to take this into account. Not any longer: We now have a single measure, no allowance for sex or age. If you want to avoid using the BMI ratio you would be in good company. **Many now regard the simple waist measurement as a more reliable way to forecast disasters ahead**. A report by the *World Health Organization* suggests increased risk when the waist measurement exceeds 37 inches (94cm) for men or 32 inches (80cm) for women.

A more sophisticated way of assessing the amount and distribution of internal fat, ideally less than 2 litres, is unlikely to become popular because it requires MRI scans. The BMI is still widely used so details are on the Table. Between 20 and 25 is normal. Below 20 is the realm of the undernourished, the anorexic, fashion models and ambitious jockeys. Above 25 is overweight, above 30 obese; above 40 morbid obesity, which requires urgent action. Most of us will have some idea what weight we would like to be. Using the chart can help, but choose a target within reach rather than a theoretical ideal. The midpoint of normal, 22.5, the theoretically average desirable weight, could be your target but we still need to consider individual variations of shape – stocky, wiry and so forth. The principle of moderation means not aiming as low as 20, the boundary of the anorexic.

'Experts' tell us to avoid setting a target fearing we should become obsessed. This is irrelevant for normal people. It is common sense to choose your target, even if it involves a more modest weight loss than advised by the table. Others tell us not to weigh regularly in case we become upset by day-to-day variations; some believe weighing-scales should be banished completely, sensible perhaps for psychiatric patients or the irrational, but for the rest of us it is logical to keep an eye on progress by regular or occasional weighing as the individual wants. Occasional variations don't matter; choosing the same time of day will help to reduce these. The natural tendency is for weight loss to taper off as the ideal weight is approached; it is often difficult to get rid of the last few pounds.

Table of weights & different heights (imperial measurements) for 5 Key BMI numbers: (3 Normal levels plus Obesity and Morbid Obesity level)

Height	BMI 20	BMI 22.5	BMI 25	BMI 30	BMI 40
Ft In	Low Normal	Mid Normal	High Normal	Obesity Level	Morbid Obesity
4' 10"	6 st 12 lb	7 st 9 lb	8 st 7 lb	10 st 3 lb	13 st 9 lb
4' 11"	7 st 1 lb	8 st 0 lb	8 st 12 lb	10 st 8 lb	14 st 2 lb
5' 0"	7 st 4 lb	8 st 3 lb	9 st 2 lb	10 st 13 lb	14 st 9 lb
5' 1"	7 st 8 lb	8 st 7 lb	9 st 6 lb	11 st 4 lb	15 st 2 lb
5' 2"	7 st 11 lb	8 st 11 lb	9 st 10 lb	11 st 10 lb	15 st 9 lb
5' 3"	8 st 1 lb	9 st 1 lb	10 st 1 lb	12 st 1 lb	16 st 2 lb
5' 4"	8 st 4 lb	9 st 5 lb	10 st 5 lb	12 st 6 lb	16 st 9lb
5' 5"	8 st 8 lb	9 st 9 lb	10 st 10 lb	12 st 12 lb	17 st 2 lb
5' 6"	8 st 12 lb	9 st 13 lb	10 st 13 lb	13 st 4 lb	17 st 10 lb
5' 7"	9 st 1 lb	10 st 3 lb	11 st 5 lb	13 st 9 lb	18 st 3 lb
5' 8"	9 st 5 lb	10 st 7 lb	11 st 10 lb	14 st 1 lb	18 st 11 lb
5' 9"	9 st 9 lb	10 st 12 lb	12 st 1 lb	14 st 7 lb	19 st 5 lb
5' 10"	9 st 13 lb	11 st 2 lb	12 st 6 lb	14 st 11 lb	19 st 13 lb
5' 11"	10 st 3 lb	11 st 7 lb	12 st 11lb	15 st 5 lb	20 st 7 lb
6' 0"	10 st 7 lb	11 st 11 lb	13 st 2 lb	15 st 11 lb	21 st 1 lb
6' 1"	10 st 12 lb	12 st 2 lb	13 st 7 lb	16 st 3 lb	21 st 9lb
6' 2"	11 st 2 lb	12 st 7 lb	13 st 13 lb	16 st 10 lb	22 st 4 lb
6' 3 "	11 st 6 lb	12 st 12 lb	14 st 4 lb	17 st 2 lb	22 st 12 lb
6' 4"	11 st 10 lb	13 st 2 lb	14 st 9 lb	17 st 8 lb	23 st 7 lb
6' 5"	12 st 1 lb	13 st 8 lb	15 st 1 lb	18 st 1 lb	24 st 1 lb
6' 6"	12 st 5 lb	13 st 13 lb	15 st 6 lb	18 st 7 lb	24 st 10 lb
6' 7"	12 st 9 lb	14 st 4 lb	15 st 12 lb	19 st 0 lb	25 st 5 lb

Body Mass Index is Weight in kg divided by square of height in metres

To calculate it in imperial units:

Weight in pounds, multiplied by 703, divided by square of height in inches.

BMI is normal between 20 and 25; Between 25 and 30 is "overweight";

Over 30: "Obesity" – Over 40: "Morbid Obesity".

Note: Morbid Obese level figures are double those in the low normal range;

BMI is related to the square of your height.

The "normal" weight can differ (BMI 20 -25) for each height by as much as 1 st 9 lbs (ht 4' 10") to 3 st 3 lbs (ht 6' 7"),

This allows scope to choose your own target

Letter 3: Initial problems

Dear H

Conventional diets are incompatible with normal life. They fail because, 1) they ignore individual responsibility, 2) designed for a theoretical average they are unsuitable for most who need to lose weight; 3) most are aimed at people needing, or already under psychiatric care; few cater for normal people. 4) They make no allowance for individual quirks.

Each of us is different, so we cannot guess the quantities, or how narrow the range might be between the amount of food needed for gain and how small is the amount needed for loss, or how wide the range might be that gives stability. Only trial and error can teach this. Because we all are different, it is absurd to try and calculate calorie needs. Even if we knew our metabolic rate, change in dietary intake would soon alter it; a reduction in intake slows metabolism, so organizing a diet on calorie calculation is likely to fail. It provides a spurious impression of scientific validity – a waste of time. The simple strategy of eating less focuses on eating habits; the aim is to prevent self-absorption about eating.

When you accept that eating more than you need is the reason **you** are overweight, it follows that the only way you can lose weight is to eat less than needed. It must be less than current consumption; how much less, you decide. We each react differently when intake is reduced. Until you see how you react, decide by trial and error. It is imperative for you to make the decisions, guided by advice (not orders), common sense and your own growing experience. The rigorous control of quantity applies while reducing weight. How long this first stage lasts depends on whether you opt for a short sharp loss, or a more gradual steady one; it also depends on the amount normally eaten and on how much weight is to be shed.

How much less to start with? It depends on how quick a result is wanted. A suggestion, not an order: Try halving the normal amount and see what happens. The quantity each of us eats varies enormously, so it is impossible to forecast how each will react. Some will need to halve again before weight is shed. Reduce yet again if necessary. The second principle of moderation means no starvation or excessive exercise; this complies with the third principle of common sense. Ignore advice conflicting with either.

Diets prescribed as suitable for all, are expensive; eating less than usual, will reduce living costs. Contrast this with clothes: individually tailored cost more than ready-made. If you need to postpone rigorous weight loss for any reason – social, holiday commitments or simply because you feel like it – remember at least to avoid going back to the food intake that caused the problem. The sooner you become accustomed to eating less the easier it will be to start changing eating habits for the rest of your life. Practicing reduced food intake during Stage One should be welcomed as a learning experience as we discover how smaller quantities can satisfy and be enjoyed! There is no alternative to a rigorous regime while shedding weight.

Many with dietary problems – gluten intolerance or diabetes, for example – accept without question the necessity of radical permanent change of eating habits. It is curious that those who need to change theirs because of weight problems are resentful and reluctant to do so. Where is their gratitude for their good fortune – their double good fortune? They are free of disease and they live in an affluent environment where choice of food is enormous, while so many elsewhere cope with famine, starvation and poverty.

Letter 4: How to eat less

Dear H

*For those aiming to lose weight, the instruction "Eat less", however unwelcome, is expected. An edict that could come from Whitehall, as it did in the days of rationing, is not advice many would buy. It is counterbalanced by another instruction, one that cannot be imagined coming from Whitehall, nor from the slimming industry: Eat what **you** like. This revolutionary liberating advice does not conflict with the terse instruction "Eat less"; the balanced combination of the two interdependent messages is vital for successful weight loss.*

The advice to eat less is not always easy to follow though most people who try, manage to interpret the instructions well enough to lose weight. If the first attempt does not work, eat yet less again.

Often we need to eat what is put before us, though our preference might be different, either because the family eats together, or we eat socially with others. No one else can solve this problem. Whether you postpone weight loss for another day or week, or are firm and risk social embarrassment, is for you to decide. For those who prepare their own meals this difficulty will be less, but it will often obtrude if social life is busy.

What we eat has a direct link to becoming overweight. Ridding ourselves of the excess is the aim of Stage One. To do this you restrict intake, by voluntary individual choices, the rigour and severity of which you decide for yourself. In Stage Two, to prevent the weight coming back, you must accept there is no alternative to changing your eating habits.

When the target weight is achieved, celebration is appropriate, but restrained to avoid relapse. After completing the difficult part: semi-starving to burn off the excess fat, it would be stupid not to change your habits to prevent the problem recurring. Many believe it is impossible to lose weight by controlling food intake. They deny eating more than they need. The reasons given are rationalizations or excuses. They claim they have no self-control, or alternatively if weight is lost, it is sure to be quickly regained.

There is a valid equation between intake and weight gain and loss; but it is different for each of us. Everyone can lose weight by eating less. The brutal fact is there was no obesity in concentration camps. Involuntary restriction of food, for example natural calamities, shipwreck, imprisonment by hostage takers, mountaineering catastrophes – all teach the same lesson. A modern equivalent, the 'health farm', operates on the same principle of forcible restriction of intake, an extreme and expensive way of dealing with the aim to lose weight. The 'health farm' offers little or no help in the difficult problem of preventing the regaining of weight when liberty is restored. As we shall see in Letter 11, compassionate starvation can cure even morbid obesity, when allied to a determination to change eating habits.

It is patronizing and foolish to assume what suits one will be right for everyone. A prescribed diet, theoretically correct for a hypothetical average, will not help many normal people. On an identical regime, some will gain weight, some will remain steady and other will lose weight. The fact that some gained weight in the Surrey Diet Trials (see Letter 19) came as a surprise to its organizers. It was predictable.

Letter 5: Moderation and Common Sense

Dear H

'He had the good sense to . . ' implies more than cleverness or knowledge; it means he had common sense, sense of perspective, and judgment. In fact he had wisdom. Richard Asher, Physician (1912-1969)

You can maintain a steady weight, at the chosen level, eating less than those around you. Eat what you want; the Choice is open - it is wide. Enjoy it. The limit is the portion size. Common sense and will power is vital for this decision. You must do it yourself. DIY. No one else can. When celebrating or if for any reason you eat more than planned, compensate for it later by a self-chosen restriction.

Reducing intake to zero might seem logical for quick weight loss. Many have tried; it is neither moderate nor sensible. Starvation is a viable exceptional option for morbid obesity for example but without supervision complications can be horrendous. Missing an occasional meal, is no great harm; many find it a convenient way to reduce intake, but it should be an occasional meal missed, not successive ones. Those who starve unsupervised become self-absorbed; mental problems follow, anorexia, bulimia; associated problems of food addiction, induced vomiting and denial. Psychiatric treatment is needed but is not always successful.

The idea of 'being on a diet for the rest of your life' is a negative reaction. The fear of it is often cited for refusing to try this Plan. This is the view of a pessimist. A diet is a prescribed course of food regime. The significant point is that someone else prescribes it; the client (victim) is reduced to obeying orders. Be positive and look at our advantages. No foods are forbidden, restrictions are self-chosen. The range available is enlarged, with a common sense limitation of the total amount. Using common sense is easier, and more satisfying, than accepting unreasonable edicts from impersonal authority figures.

Having full control of your choice of menus, how you arrange the details is up to you. Your meals will be more adventurous and enjoyable. Counteract the disadvantage of being careful about total quantities by enjoying the novelty of unfamiliar food, while not forgetting old favourites.

Not all of us need to lose weight. About half the population has the tendency to store fat rather than burn it up: it is their inheritance; it is genetic. Those affected have the "fat" gene; it is familial though not all are equally burdened. We with the inborn tendency to store fat must accept the link between what we eat and what we store. The remedy is in our hands: waste no time envying those who never gain weight however much they eat; they may be in the same families as those affected by the "fat" gene, yet despite the same upbringing they stay thin. We with the "fat" gene might resent the unfairness of life, but should not dwell on our misfortune. Life is unfair; we must accept our lot.

A lesson from children: competitiveness when eating. Watch them when food is being served: although they keep an eye on what goes on their own plate, they watch with greater intensity what others are given. If asked how much they would like, the answer is likely to be 'my fair share'. In the animal kingdom we are familiar with vivid images of chicks fed by a mother bird, with the weakest allowed to starve; this is not paralleled in civilized human behaviour. We must abandon the ingrained feeling that we deserve our 'fair share'; some need more than others in the family.

Letter 6: Eating Habits and Food Fads

Dear H

The need to change our eating habits is unwelcome; most of us resist change. It is a common reason for refusing even to consider trying a weight reduction programme. Having learnt it is possible to reduce food intake it is sensible, indeed imperative to go one step further. Make the change permanent.

Too often battles about food with small children end with bargaining about how much must be eaten to satisfy honour on both sides – the origin of many irrational food fads, which persist long after the original battle has been forgotten. Mature adults should extend the range of what they eat, keep the amount small and learn to enjoy eating less.

Not being on a diet we can delight in the challenge of new foods. Learn to enjoy them and the chance of trying new tastes. Revisit the fads and dislikes accumulated since childhood. It is never too late to discard them. However these irrational dislikes arise, we all have them. Being irrational they should disappear from our new schedule. It is sensible to look at them afresh as we grow older and hopefully wiser, especially when embarking on a new way of watching what we eat. Many foods we refuse are popular with others, often bland in taste; indeed we eat them without qualms when they occur in other recipes. A long-standing dislike of a particular food is not a good reason for still refusing to eat it. Give it a try, perhaps by blind tasting as a sign of maturity and common sense.

Many eating habits are established in infancy, though the initial diet was breast milk or a prepared supplement; once solids are introduced, any time after the first few weeks, the infant will unmistakably express approval or distaste for anything unfamiliar.

The new mother of a first-born is as much a beginner as the child. If she is apprehensive or tentative, the infant soon realises it can decide when food should be offered and if it is what it wants. Success in imposing its will becomes a habit, entrenched as the infant discovers its new power. The combination of an uncertain mother and a demanding infant is a recipe for a spoilt child; in the opposite situation, a placid undemanding amenable infant with a confident or experienced mother produces a child who quickly learns what is acceptable behaviour. With so many variables for both mother and infant between the two scenarios, there is a predictably large variety of response by infants when offered food.

The earliest battle for a small child is usually about food. A firm parent – it can be a father or a mother – decides to impose a particular item; the opening skirmish begins if the child refuses it. The scene can develop in many ways, but a determined child, 'obstinate' in the parent's view, has the advantage. The sensible strategy is to avoid a battle; too often an over-confident or obstinate parent provokes a disastrous and unnecessary confrontation. Ideally the parent should be firm, but a child quickly senses when it has the upper hand. A battle won or lost can imprint the beginning of a food fad.

Other fads come with school meals. The fashionable wide choice encourages them. This over-generous provision encourages children to believe they have the right to pick and choose. To offer young children a choice of food, unheard of in the Third World, unavailable in most countries, before they are qualified to make a rational choice, is foolish. The agenda for school meals, the emphasis on children's rights, and choice firmly embedded, all encourage food fads. The signal is that children have the right to choose unsuitable food as often as they like.

Letter 7: Our Digestive Tract

"The growth of knowledge depends entirely on disagreement"

(Karl R. Popper 1902-1994)

Dear H

*When self-styled nutritionists, supported by the Department of Health, tell us 'we are what we eat', we should remember Karl Popper's dictum and disagree. We are **not** what we eat. We are what we create from what we eat. This depends on instructions from our genetic codes. Some of us are programmed to construct and store fat more readily than others – this is not from fat ingested, but from what we ourselves make.*

During the last century the prevailing dogma, universally accepted, was that bacteria could not survive in the stomach because it was so highly acidic. Australian doctors Warren and Marshall challenged this in 1984, claiming a bacterium as a cause of peptic ulcer. They were attacked for questioning the wisdom of their superiors. Pharmaceutical companies hastened to defend their ulcer-healing drugs with numerous 'expert' opinions. It was not until Marshall swallowed the bacterium responsible and produced an ulcer that a sceptical medical profession reluctantly accepted this new fact. Fortunately an antibiotic cured it but it was a further ten years before most doctors embraced the new treatment. A Nobel Prize awarded in 2005 acknowledged not only Warren and Marshall's historic discovery but also their tenacity and determination in persevering with their research.

Ignorance about the basic physiology of our digestive tracts is nothing to be ashamed of – most car drivers don't know how the internal combustion engine works, computer users have no idea how computer programs work. Stories about 'unhealthy fats' or cholesterol entering the blood stream from the stomach are nonsense. The stomach is an acidic cauldron into which food enters after leaving the gullet. The contents, whether refined or coarse, are soon rendered unrecognisable. This can be deduced by common sense: anybody who has vomited knows it. Regrettably this evidence is visible in many of our town centres when the pubs close. Nutritionists appearing on TV have the effrontery to remove and throw away items from the fridges of the obese because they are 'junk food'. It might be 'good television' but it is poor science.

Everything we eat is changed by our digestive tract into basic units. From these each of us constructs what the body needs, depending on genetic instructions. Complex carbohydrates are broken down into the basic glucose. Fats, whether saturated or unsaturated, from high or low quality origin, dairy, organic, all are reduced to basic units (lipo-proteins), from which each of us constructs what we are programmed to make. Proteins, whether from expensive organic meat, or from cheaper cuts and from vegetable proteins, are all reduced to the basic amino acids, from which our robust and versatile digestive system assembles in its factory what is needed.

This is **not** the message from nutritionists or from the DoH, and if the simplified account in the paragraphs above is accurate, the implications are profound. We cannot trust current propaganda about healthy and unhealthy foods; nor can we believe eating the wrong sort of food causes obesity. Eating foods with high fat content or rich in cholesterol is not relevant to our blood fat or cholesterol levels.

Paracelsus (1493-1541) told us 500 years ago. *"Everything is harmful, and nothing is non-harmful; only the dosage makes it safe.*

Letter 8: Experts

Dear H

"An expert is one who has made every conceivable mistake within a very narrow field" *Niels Bohr, physicist*

What happens when expert opinions are diametrically opposed? Both cannot be right. They may both be wrong. For every expert opinion in favour of any dotty proposition, a number of other expert opinions can be mustered to support an alternative, whether sensible or even dottier. Critical common sense analysis is needed.

A relevant example is John Yudkin, renowned in the 1950s for his work on glucose metabolism and diabetes. His reputation suffered after he described carbohydrates as nutritionally worthless. Some years later his dietary advice became the basis for the Atkins Diet; it is instructive and salutary to see why and how a 'conceivable' mistake occurred. Yudkin noted that many overweight and obese had abnormal glucose metabolism. He concluded this was a significant cause of obesity, ignoring a more sensible alternative: it could be a result of obesity, not the cause. Atkins later based his diet on the same fallacy. These were the critical moments when complicated and erroneous dietary schemes were erected on shaky foundations.

Other eminent experts vigorously oppose the low-carbohydrate schemes of Yudkin, Atkins and the more recent Montignac; they claim the way to solve the ever-increasing epidemic of obesity and associated health problems is to return to eating plenty of starchy, unprocessed cereals and grains. Rural African tribes with diets based on grain (millet, sorghum, maize), fruit and vegetables, and sour milk, do not develop heart disease, stroke, or most cancers. Nor are they obese. In 19th-century Ireland the population subsisted largely on potatoes – until the crop failed. Famine followed; the survivors emigrated to the USA where their descendants are now obese.

Other arguments against Atkins are explored in Letter 19. Despite the popularity of Atkins, for thirty years his diet failed to dent the relentless rise in obesity either in the USA where the diet first became fashionable or elsewhere. But as to the alternative view, whatever the merits of starchy unprocessed cereals, it is unrealistic to expect the affluent to revert to a Third World diet.

Nutritionists with modest expertise also provide absurd results. *The British Medical Journal* recounts a trial of obesity in primary care (8/11/03). They evaluated 635 patients from 44 general practices over several years to see how a training programme (4 or 5 hours) on weight management advocating lifestyle change could help. The result was ludicrous: the staff acquired a better knowledge of weight management strategies but no patients lost weight. Nor did nutritionists have much success with volunteers in the Surrey University Diet Trials (see Letter 19). Only 17 out of 300 (less than 6%) achieved the modest target – a 10% reduction in their Body Mass Index in six months. These individuals showed initiative, being successful despite the advisers. Both studies caused a mountain of paperwork – graphs, statistics, analysis and discussions; bureaucracy stultifies anything it touches. More recently Dr Ben Goldacre in his best seller *Bad Science* (2009) devastatingly describes the deficiencies of nutritionists in general and one in particular.

Expert opinions are distrusted with good reason; they are often contradictory. When experts cannot agree about treatment or causes we must use common sense. A third way, the way of moderation advocated here, is preferable.

Letter 9: Causes of Obesity

Dear H

"I see ordinarily that men, when facts are put before them, are more ready to amuse themselves by inquiring into their reasons than by inquiring into their truth." Michel Montaigne (1533-1592)

The obesity crisis is not because some eat too much fat, or others eat too many carbohydrates. It is because we all eat more than we need. This is the prime significant immediate cause of being overweight or obese. When the whole population overeats, half or more will be affected. The 'epidemic' of untreatable obesity is the inevitable consequence.

Asking experts the cause of obesity produces bewildering different opinions. A physician believes it is due to a metabolic disorder, not an eating one. Psychiatrists opt for addiction to food, or lack of self-esteem. A nutritionist lists foods to be forbidden. A geriatrician recommends banning many things so as to prolong life – life expectancy would probably be unchanged but life would seem longer. A paediatrician tells us the foods children should avoid; child psychologists how they should choose for themselves. Department of Health officials tell us how much alcohol, fat, sugar, pieces of fruit or food traffic-lighted green should be eaten, advice notoriously ignored.

Dr Nikhil Dhurandhar argues that a human adenovirus, Ad-36, could be responsible for the explosion of obesity; even if true, this has no immediate relevance. Possible vaccination is a long way off. Virologists, reluctant to blame one of their viruses, believe there are simpler explanations. Epidemiologists recognise the link with affluence. Other relevant factors, upbringing, familial customs, eating habits, size of portions, snacking and the types of food involved, especially the fat-laden ones are endlessly analysed. Compounding the problem, the food industry and its advertising accomplices encourage us all to eat more than we need.

Some 'causes' associated with the rise in obesity are consequences of obesity rather than causes. (See Letter 8). Michel Montignac, promoting a recent French variant of the Atkins Diet, has followed Yudkin and Atkins by blaming a dysfunctional pancreas. He blames it for inability to deal with glucose produced by the 'wrong' carbohydrates we all eat, including potato. The dysfunctional pancreas he diagnoses in the overweight as the cause of obesity is a consequence of overloading the digestive system. This he describes as the cause, but ignores the probability of it being a result of obesity He introduced the *Glycaemic Index* (GI) to tell us which carbohydrates are most quickly metabolized. But carbohydrates like sucrose are transformed automatically into glucose. The GI might interest diabetics but they have managed very well without it.

What is the true cause? Weight has increased in step with affluence both here and in the USA. Eating more than we need stands out as the prime significant immediate cause, with eating habits and snacking as important contributory factors; all are reversible if we are willing to act.

Failure happens because too many have abandoned moderation in food consumption. Surrendering their independence they are willing accomplices in a farcical charade, unable to reverse their tragic role, yo-yoing between weight loss and weight gain. Listen to advice, but when experts disagree use common sense.

The difficulty confronting each of us will vary, but we must try. Though not easy to lose weight, it is possible. Christianity was said to be impossible to practise because it had been tried and found wanting. G. K. Chesterton said the truth was that it had been found difficult and not tried. So with weight loss: difficult to achieve, but not impossible. It varies for each of us but it is often much easier than expected.

Letter 10: 50 Years Increase in Obesity

Dear H

Fifty years ago obesity was rare. There has been a steady increase in the numbers of people overweight since then. Appeals to eat sensibly are ignored.

We need only look at old news reels to see how uncommon obesity was, especially during and for some years after the 1939-1945 war when food was rationed. The impression is confirmed by seeing what happens in the USA where obesity is even more of a problem than here, clearly linked to the enormous portions served in USA restaurants and homes.

The worldwide increase in people both overweight (BMI 25-30) and obese (BMI over 30) has been apparent for many years, and is approaching danger levels. In the USA it is suggested that those responsible for the increase in ill-health be called to account; restaurants and food advertisers should be prosecuted, just as the tobacco industry is being held responsible for cigarette-related deaths and illnesses.

Recently the Worldwatch Institute in Washington estimated 1.2 billion is the number of people overweight (BMI over 25) in the world; since then it is larger than those who are malnourished, hungry and underfed (BMI under 20). The proportion of overweight people (BMI over 25) is highest in the USA (55%). Over ten years, figures for the UK have increased by 10% to 51% so we are catching up. Even in China, not yet an affluent society, the percentage has jumped from 9% to 15% in three years. Obesity (BMI over 30) in the UK has risen from 7% in 1980 to 18% in 1997, and is now about the same as in the USA.

Clearly there is a public health problem. The failure of authority to protect us from hazards such as drug addiction and smoking gives little confidence they will succeed in tackling the problem of an overweight population. Individuals must concentrate on the simple strategy of eating less.

Statistics are used to prove anything, but it is difficult to imagine a more contentious use of figures to construct a false theory, while claiming to dismiss pseudo-science, than Montignac's argument (using WHO study figures) that a 30-35% decrease in calories consumed in the West in the last 50 years has been matched with a 400% rise in obesity, most alarmingly among young children. We all know there has been no decrease in calories consumed; they have steadily risen. The WHO figures are wrong or quoted out of context, yet Montignac says *"forget calorie control; the rise in obesity is to do with eating the wrong food, not eating too many calories."* The opposite is true.

We become obese by eating too much. Anyone with common sense knows this. Ask the man in the street. The human digestive system (see Letter 7) is robust and versatile; it copes with the extraordinary variety of substances we inflict on it. The affluent expect it to cope with excesses; rarely is it defeated. What it cannot digest it will try and store; it will excrete what it cannot use. When grossly overloaded it is perverse and illogical to blame its occasional failure as the cause of obesity when it is the consequence.

Letter 11: Morbid Obesity

Dear H

The small but growing numbers who suffer from Morbid Obesity (BMI over 40) present a most challenging problem, their situation is life-threatening; help is needed urgently. Some sufferers have benefited from advice in this Plan; it will suit others, especially those with a less serious weight problem.

Most sufferers from Morbid Obesity have tried many remedies without success. They have become depressed with repeated failure. Exhortations to take more exercise are heartless and inappropriate. They carry a physical burden few thin people would contemplate lifting. The energy expended in moving about is much more than the heaviest exercise schedule to which keen fitness fanatics would submit. This increases their desire for food. Trapped in a truly vicious circle they deserve compassion, not criticism, sympathy and understanding, not ostracism. Their plight is compounded by the false belief that their metabolic rate is too low to burn up their fat. In reality many, especially the more active, have a high metabolic rate, needed to sustain the enormous burden they carry. Only when swimming can they compete on equal terms with those of normal weight. Immersion in water lifts the burden; one indomitable group has demonstrated grace and ability by indulging in fashionable synchronized swimming.

How to treat this condition is problematic; they are all different, the solution for one is not right for another. The morbid obese are also subject to the laws of physics. Robust effective treatment including starvation for a desperate exceptional condition means moderation takes a lower priority.

A GP colleague in Bristol proved this nearly 50 years ago, when he admitted patients to GP beds for a fortnight, most referred by fellow GPs, to prove to each, that despite their fixed belief they could not lose weight, he guaranteed each would lose at least one stone in the two weeks. Over ten years, at least a hundred such patients were so treated; they all lost over the stone promised. The regime was starvation for one week with fluids only and in the second week small portions of fish, chicken and vegetables. One patient went on to lose a further seven stone after discharge, an example of morbid obesity successfully treated by compassionate starvation. At this time surgeons were wiring jaws or removing ileums. Current surgical treatment – bypassing the stomach and gut, removing aprons of fat, is equally radical. It says more for the compassion and courage of a surgeon prepared to do this than for his sagacity. Organised starvation is surely preferable to heroic surgery. Could this be done now?

A similar experiment is unlikely; few GPs have access to NHS beds, or time from form-filling to alleviate obesity so economically; ward sisters able to impose the necessary discipline no longer exist; few patients would submit to such a spartan regime; a hospital authority would fear being sued for infringement of human rights. Instead we have the ludicrous pathetic spectacle of those with morbid obesity, trapped at home, too bulky even to get out of bed, with no hope of ever leaving their room, yet meals on wheels are delivered regularly, aggravating their situation.

Some indomitable and determined patients can and do change their eating habits and become thin; there is always hope others will follow, despite the exceptional difficulties to be overcome. Hope must never be abandoned.

Letter 12: Will exercise make us healthy?

Dear H

To rely on exercise to reduce weight is to court disappointment. Restricting food intake is more efficient. Exercise should be moderate, and postponed if it causes discomfort or breathlessness. Ambitious exercise programmes are often an excuse for eating more than we know we should. The hope of burning off significant amounts of fat by exercise is illusory. The amount of physical effort needed to counteract food bingeing is far greater than those trying to control their weight by reduced intake can manage.

Fitness fanatics urge us to take more exercise. The chap, who whenever he was tempted to exercise, lay down until the urge passed, represents the opposite view. Committed to moderation, we listen to extremists carefully, and are wary of their advice. We should be moderate in exercising; though it helps to burn up fat, it also increases appetite; this in turn makes us eat more. Weight gained will not be balanced by weight burned off by exercise. To burn off one pound of fat, you need to walk 35 miles.

Losing weight it is said to make us fitter and/or healthier. An American cardiologist, Henry Solomon, in *The Exercise Myth*, (1984), emphasised that the fad current then – it still persists – for expensive gym exercise treatment and 'workouts' is based on the fallacy that fitness and health are equivalent. This is not so. Fitness is a measure of how well the body can perform physical tasks. It is a measure of the greatest amount of oxygen the body can use when performing at peak effort. It is possible to be physically fit, yet fatally ill with coronary heart disease, as the fate of some joggers has demonstrated.

Conversely one can be wonderfully healthy, but unfit in terms of exercise capacity. Health is largely determined by our genetic inheritance, though modified by life style. Too much unsuitable exercise can be dangerous; jogging can aggravate arthritic hips, knees and ankles. It is absurd to spend time and money, on unnecessary equipment, when walking is an ideal and safe alternative. Criticism from an all-party committee of MPs that the Government has been scandalously remiss in not instituting a Walking Strategy for us all is inept. Individuals should decide whether or not to walk for exercise.

Some enjoy exercising while others are less enthusiastic. It is sensible is to do as much or as little as one prefers; there should be no pressure on the reluctant merely because the current fashion is for 'exercise centres' and 'working out', an option notably absent in less affluent societies. It is difficult to believe some joggers really enjoy their activity judging by their expressions of pain and distress; jogging to exhaustion produces endorphins in the blood stream, related to break down of opiates; the jogger achieves a heroin-like effect; the suffering involved is preferable to dependence on a drug supplier. It is also cheaper and safer.

Advice to exercise ignores the fact that many so advised are trapped in a vicious circle starting with inertia, due to the constant burden of carrying a load that must be shed before exercise can really begin. It is only common sense to wait until some weight is lost; the desire to exercise will return with the capacity to do so without discomfort or breathlessness. This advice may seem harsh and lacking in compassion, but it is more cruel to urge the obese, especially the young, to vigorous exercise when they carry more weight than their thin contemporaries would contemplate lifting when they exercise. I have been criticized for not emphasising the benefits of exercise. These are currently over praised elsewhere so it is necessary to redress the balance, specifically for the disabled who cannot exercise. This minority is marginalized; the message they get is that if you cannot exercise you will be unable to lose weight. Not true. Many have welcomed this assurance and have lost weight successfully.

Letter 13: Appetite and Hunger

Dear H

Breakdown of our built-in mechanism for appetite control causes many to believe that however hard they try they will never succeed in losing weight. Physical hunger responds to a small amount of food; psychological hunger can be banished by distraction.

Many fear being hungry and unable to resist food. Appetite has two elements: real physical hunger, a feeling of emptiness, and second, the craving for a particular food or flavour, both affected by psychological attitudes. The feeling of true hunger is nowadays not tolerated; craving food demands instant gratification. This is regrettable and absurd; the sense of emptiness was a normal experience until snacking became fashionable.

Learn to relish the sensation, not actually unpleasant, though now unfamiliar. Try seeing how long you can postpone eating when hungry. When you do you will realise how much better it is for you to decide when to eat.

The temptation to eat might seem irresistible yet it can be banished or postponed by distraction. An artist becomes so involved in painting that feelings of discomfort, cold, fatigue, or hunger, disappear. Any occupation or hobby will do. Conquering hunger while concentrating on something else by missing a meal can be practiced. Postponement increases the enjoyment.

Ultimately true hunger needs to be solved by food, and the feeling of emptiness disappears quickly after a few mouthfuls. If you feel you could eat a horse, you will be tempted to fill your plate with much more than you really need. Experiment and surprise yourself by how a tiny amount of food can banish the sensation of hunger. Restaurants with shameful titles like Bellybuster, advertising, "eat all you can", pander to the temptation to eat too much. Resist it.

We have become accustomed to large portions, that we feel we should eat, usually far too quickly. Second helpings are taken when not needed. There is a time-lapse between eating and the feeling of satiety; some find it helpful to try for example, a cup of tea with a little milk, drunk slowly before a meal to produce satiety earlier or perhaps an aperitif with a few nibbles.

Hunger is often a matter of habit near a mealtime but it is not a real need for food. Distinguish between degrees of hunger: they range from being absolutely ravenous to healthy hunger, fancying a nibble, comfortably full, to replete. Ignoring the two extremes, absolutely ravenous and replete, we must learn to tolerate the intermediate stages and not become obsessed by the supposed need to eat.

Eating smaller portions using simple strategies can help. Using smaller plates, or using chopsticks can encourage smaller quantities and slow eating by putting down knife and fork between mouthfuls. Many others are described in diet books but it is common sense coupled with one's own awareness that will teach us how to eat less. The more you do it, the easier it becomes. Group eating with an element of competition can increase consumption. In winter we are tempted to eat more as the body naturally tries to conserve its stores. In cold weather there is less incentive to exercise so we need to be more careful with our food intake.

Letter 14: Food Cravings

Dear H

Many believe they cannot lose weight because they succumb to food cravings. Learn to control these but do not be despondent if you do not succeed immediately. Persevere and do your best.

Can one enjoy food while losing weight? Of course! If we are not allowed to eat as much as we want, we can still enjoy favourite items. Many believe we cannot be successful unless we suffer. No foods are forbidden; we are not dieting; it is our choice to eat less than usual. Enjoy it.

Eating slowly, savouring food enhances enjoyment. The pleasure should not depend on feeling replete or bloated; small portions may not satisfy at first because we have become so accustomed to feeling full being the natural goal at the end of a meal. We should be aware and grateful that hunger has been satisfied; there is no need to feel replete. We should also extend enjoyment to more of the different types of food we choose ourselves.

Food cravings are rarely caused by a genuine physiological need for certain substances, salt or sugar for example. Choosing bananas because they are a source of potassium is not a good reason unless you also enjoy them. Most cravings are no more than whims, harmless in themselves. If we indulge these– a whim can become elevated into a belief that we really need what we want. Self-discipline is rarely practised. Indulge a passing whim; but don't use it as an excuse for eating too much.

The craving for a particular flavour can be quickly satisfied. For example chocolate: the first is delicious; the next, enjoyable. Subsequent ones are progressively more disappointing. Moderation means no more than the minimum to satisfy the craving; why eat more when enjoyment is diminishing? Postpone the next, ideally to another day. Packaging encourages us to eat more than we need. Resist this.

Snacking should be abandoned, especially while shedding weight. Common sense tells us it is foolish to indulge in calories we know we don't need; it nullifies the effect of small portions at meal times.

When your target is reached, occasional snacking is less harmful. By then most of us will have got out of the habit; don't resume it. Snacking, a regrettable part of present-day culture has become automatic when watching TV, at the cinema, or in car, coach, train, or plane when food is regularly on offer. Many suffer from snack amnesia, genuinely forgetting what they have eaten. Some inveterate snackers believe items "do not count" if they only tasted something a friend was eating. Keeping an accurate record can be next to impossible, yet some diets insist this should be done. This plan does not. If you take no snacks or 'tastes', there is no recording to be done. It is much simpler than any diet.

Letter 15: Weight loss, Reasons for and Benefits from

Dear H

Reasons to lose weight vary from the frivolous to the serious: vanity, self-esteem, to become fitter or healthier (not the same thing), or even to comply with medical advice. Benefits include increased mobility and a general feeling of well-being. Until some weight is shed few will believe how much better it is to be without this unwanted burden.

Medical advice to lose weight often given rarely followed. Problems increase with age so it is sensible to deal with it while young. Prevention is preferable to a late cure especially if it is surgical.

Many common ailments are improved by losing weight: shortness of breath, asthma, varicose veins, hernia, foot problems, arthritis, cardiac disease, diabetes and many others. They can be avoided by timely action though few embark on food restrictions to forestall possible future ill health. Non-smoking campaigns fail likewise from inertia. Motivation is the key to success.

The first benefit: satisfaction at fulfilling an ambition one had hoped to achieve for some time. Energy will return with freedom from lassitude. Few will want to return to the former state. Determination to succeed helps in sticking to the plan. Other benefits extend beyond those mentioned, relief of pain in arthritic weight-bearing joints, making stairs less of a problem, getting up from a low chair and such simple tasks as toenail cutting become easier.

The human frame functions well when burdened by excessive weight, a tribute to its design. Some cope well with an extraordinary extra burden. Suma wrestlers in Japan, enormously bulky move surprisingly nimbly; how they fare when older, or what is their life expectancy is not discussed. At the other extreme, some of us wilt when burdened by a moderate degree of excess weight. Because we all react differently to physical stress, we must allow for individual response.

Though the body adapts remarkably well, problems get worse as we grow older, and deterioration is to be expected. It is foolhardy to rely on being an exception, being: fit, fat and full of years. The sheer relief of shedding a burden carried continuously is often not anticipated, likened by some to carrying a child on each hip wherever one goes. Shedding this is equivalent to putting down a sack of potatoes. Because the burden increases gradually, it is not noticed.

Promoters of weight loss never show clients this aspect of lifting a burden, though it would be a powerful incentive. A harness, suspended from a rail, providing a variable lift factor, could show degrees of relief from various weight targets to be shed. When so much extravagant equipment is available at fashionable fitness centres, it is odd that this option is not offered.

To lose 44 lbs (20 Kg) was my target. Put in perspective, it is the luggage allowance for air travel; not a burden anyone would want to carry for long; yet many do, sometimes for years. Should we be able to negotiate a reduction of excess baggage charges on the basis of personal weight loss? Some airlines now weigh passengers as the average weight often exceeds the assumed figure considered, when balanced with fuel needs, when flights are fully booked or especially when small planes have relatively few passengers.

Letter 16: Nutrition needs and food to take with care

Dear H

Don't worry about the body's need of adequate nutrients, vitamins and minerals. Eating a healthy range of foods, including fruit and vegetables, even in small quantities it would take a near-starvation regime before any of us developed vitamin deficiency. Most populations survive on a restricted range of food yet their people get by. In affluent countries we all eat far more than we need.

On a restricted intake there will be less excreted. Provided you include fibre and adequate fluid, without which the fibre cannot do its job, this should present little difficulty. Be prepared for natural changes in your bowel habit, and welcome them. It is a sign you are making progress.

Some foods should be eaten with caution, because they are high in calories or fat. They are often described as 'junk food' (see Letter 1) and disparaged by nutritionists and the DoH who tell us to eat healthily. As our aim is to burn up stored fat, it is common sense to reduce high calorie foods. Take sufficient to make your intake palatable. Foods described as fat-free, or fat-reduced are usually also high in calories with added carbohydrates, usually sugar, to make them attractive. Take them also with caution.

What we eat is a personal choice – so no lists of food or menus! Instead some encouraging words about items likely to cause difficulties, forbidden in conventional diets, of which many of us are particularly fond: Cream and full cream milk are stigmatised as particularly bad; they are not, but the quantity taken can be too large. A small quantity of cream that is enjoyed is better than large volumes of skimmed milk that are not. Chips, confectionery, alcohol and soft drinks, all high in calories are not forbidden here but choose them occasionally and in moderate quantities. What matters is the portion size.

Choosing from menus in restaurants can be difficult. Avoid places that challenge you to eat as much as possible though it may not be your choice, but that of your host. Some venues provide smaller portions on request though not usually at a lower price. So-called children's portions though usually cheaper are not suitable for anyone wanting to eat modestly. Paradoxically it can be the most expensive places, specializing in *nouvelle cuisine*, where smaller portions are served. It goes against the grain to pay more to eat less. We can do this much better at home.

While comparatively easy to achieve balance, neither gaining nor losing weight, it is frustrating to find a period of restraint has produced no weight loss. It is impossible to predict how a particular level of intake will affect us individually. Only trial and error will teach each of us individually how much restraint is needed. The total amount is the critical factor. It is bad luck if you have to deny yourself more than others, but once you accept this, after reaching your target, you can look forward to a more generous intake without regaining weight.

If weight is not going down, there is no alternative but to cut intake, repeatedly if necessary until it does. Nobody can do this except the person concerned; that is why commercial systems aimed at the 'average' fail.

Letter 17: Will power: How much is needed?

Dear H

The answer is like the proverbial length of a piece of string: enough. Those who believe they cannot control their appetite see no point even in attempting to lose weight. They cite the lack of will power. They also believe that if they do lose weight they do not have sufficient will power to maintain this loss. If common sense does not work Psychiatric advice might help such a defeatist attitude.

Many who have clearly demonstrated their ability to control other aspects of their behaviour often use this argument, for example those who have managed to stop smoking. To be afraid of even trying to lose weight, known to be beneficial is irrational and often acknowledged as such. It is impossible to convince those who disregard rational argument. If the psychological component is amenable to reason, moderation and common sense there is hope. If irrationality persists, a psychological approach might be unavoidable.

Many schemes promoting weight loss make allowances for the irrational; most admit openly or implicitly that psychiatric considerations are of prime importance in the teaching and promotion of the particular scheme under consideration. In a recent book with the sensible though negative title, *Eating Less* (1998), Gillian Riley advocates the principle of non-dietary control by eating less. So far so good. She summarised her method in the Daily Telegraph 30/11/98, which gave similar advice to that given here. However as an expert on addiction and on smoking problems (she has published an excellent book *How to Stop Smoking and Stay Stopped for Good*), she identifies a weight problem as food addiction. This may be valid for some of her clients; and for them her detailed advice is useful. However, the proposition that we are all addicted to food is fallacious and contrary to common sense.

Her advice, targeted at the psychiatrically challenged, is not useful for and would not be accepted by the normal people at whom this present plan is aimed. Commendations of her book are from psychologists, psychotherapists and counselors. The arguments used in her book are all from that point of view. Her advice is ideal for those with addictive personalities and those receiving psychiatric treatment. Normal people resist referral to a psychiatrist – 'I haven't come to that yet, doctor' is a common reaction. Her advice that self-esteem should be the target, rather than weight loss, is as unacceptable as that weighing scales should be banned. The normal reject advice given from a psychiatric point of view, yet those who have the temerity to challenge these interpretations are stigmatised as being 'in denial'.

Advice, sensible for a normal person, has to be disguised for those with psychiatric problems, either by role-play or equivalent to make it work. The problem of dealing with psychiatric patients is their irrationality and inability to use common sense. The question of food addiction, claimed by some psychiatrists to be at the root of most eating problems, is considered in Letter 20.

Weight Matters for Young People by Dr Rachel Pryke (2006) provides comprehensive sensible up-to-date information for a generation who might find the advice here impractical.

18: Some older diets and their problems

Dear H

Considering the enormous variety of foods consumed in many parts of the world, in different presentations, it is astonishing how adaptable our digestive tract is in coping with this wide range of food. It copes with the unsuitable. (See Letter 7). There is no need to pander to a supposed need of detoxification. Though used by the affluent, the poor scorn it. Diets based on dubious theories should be avoided, for example those forbidding eating proteins and carbohydrates together.

From the enormous number of remedies for obesity only a few can be considered. The four most popular in the UK are discussed in Letter 19.

Different dietary systems have waxed and waned over the last half century. In my early years in general practice in the late forties and fifties, food rationing, imposed during the 1939-45 war, was being gradually relaxed; obesity was rare and of little concern. Since then it has been an increasing problem.

In the fifties and sixties John Yudkin and followers promoted low-carbohydrate and high-protein diets. Carbohydrates were "nutritionally useless, sugars positively harmful" (see letter 8). In the USA those overweight were described as allergic to carbohydrates, with overproduction of insulin. Any success from diets prescribed then was due to restricted daily intake and fewer calories. In the sixties and seventies, more people became overweight as food consumption increased with affluence. Amphetamines and other appetite suppressants became popular, each with their own specific disadvantages, as modern drugs still have.

For those seeking quick results the *Beverly Hills Diet* claimed pineapple would burn away fat; others advocated grapes and little else; marginally more attractive was the odd combination of eggs and grapefruit. The monotony of those regimes meant few could stick them for long. *The Scarsdale Medical Diet*, a strict 14-day 1000-calorie high-protein plan gave dramatic losses, but caused muscle and bone depletion as well as the desired fat loss. When normal eating was resumed muscles and bone recovered, and the fat returned.

In the eighties high fibre was advocated, carbohydrates returned to favour, especially the potato. *The F-Plan* was an early best seller, still popular, promoting bread and cereals. At the same time the *Hip and Thigh Diet* (Rosemary Conley) emphasised foods to be forbidden. Its claim to remove fat from specific parts of the body was never proved. A later version is one of the four considered in the next letter. Quick fixes like the *Cabbage Soup Diet* included such quirks as single foods on some days, bananas or steak to counter monotony, as supplements to limitless cabbage soup. Reduced calorie intake from these regimes was achieved and it is still marketed with up to 5 variants, ranging from 400 to 1500 calories daily. *Detoxification Diets* claimed to remove poisons allegedly present in processed and refined foods. These were forbidden. The poisons "could only be reversed by 'natural' foods" – a proposition lacking credible evidence.

In the nineties the *Hay Diet*, popular 100 years ago, reappeared, claiming protein and carbohydrate were incompatible and should not be mixed at the same meal – not credible from common sense or with the explosion in popularity of sandwiches. *The Hay Diet* cuts fat; any success is from low calorie intake. *Low-fat diets*, then fashionable, became more complicated with arguments about the merits or dangers of saturated and unsaturated fats and worries about cholesterol levels. 'Experts' worry again about carbohydrates, whether we eat the right kind, or their effect on insulin levels, just as they did forty years ago. Schemes advertised on TV, in newspapers, magazines and books depend ultimately on reducing intake, implying it can be done without discomfort. The rules are impossibly rigid for anyone living a normal working life – weighing what you eat, counting calories, with protein and fat, subdivided into separate categories: proteins into different amino-acids, fats into saturated and unsaturated and whichever of these is believed not to increase cholesterol levels. Carbohydrates are recurrently in and out of fashion; potatoes, condemned as bad, have now become good. Shopping for suitable foods can be a nightmare for those foolish enough to believe those who tell us how to choose healthy foods. Contradictory and incompatible arguments abound; sensible people ignore them and eat what they enjoy in modest quantities.

Then there are those forbidden foods. Forbidding something makes it more desirable. *Slimmers World* recognises this classifying their forbidden foods as 'sins', allowing a limited number. Though better than an outright ban, it is not a sensible answer. The compilers of such lists don't have the competence to decide what anyone else should eat, or which should be forbidden. We must recover responsibility for what we will eat and what we will not.

Anti-obesity drugs are unsatisfactory, side effects, failure to produce weight loss reliably, and serious problems such as addiction; if they work, the response is uncertain and often fleeting. Those who become addicted to such drugs have the worst possible outcome: a sad drug-dependent individual, still overweight, with the maladies associated with obesity compounded by the new problem of addiction. Most people who need to lose weight can do it themselves if encouraged to adopt a simple regime of eating less. Many convincing examples of permanently maintained weight loss are from individuals who have devised their own regimes. We should follow their example.

Letter 19: Uncontrolled Obesity

Dear H

Options for the overweight have been (a) to follow advice from the Department of Health using an approved slimming regime: low fat, cholesterol, salt and calorie intake, or (b) to try a fashionable cranky alternative, the most popular recently being the Atkins Diet forbidding carbohydrates. None has halted the steady rise of obesity. In an affluent society with all eating more than we need, imposing an unacceptable regime is a fundamental flaw of officially approved diets. Individuals are not encouraged to use a simple non-dietary method yet everyone would lose weight efficiently, cheaply, and successfully maintain the loss, eating less of what they like and not what someone else tells them.

The University of Surrey supervised a 6-month trial (ending April '03) to identify the best of the four most popular (and profitable) schemes used in the UK: *Slimfast, Rosemary Conley, Weight Watchers* and the *Dr Atkins New Diet*. 300 volunteers were randomly assigned to these four. It was naïve to expect to find 'the best'. The result: 17 out of 300 – less than 6%, lost weight, unrelated to the method each used. There was no clear winner from the four plans.

Slimfast, with meal replacement by milk-shakes, soups, or pasta for two of three main meals, is simple to follow, often wilfully misinterpreted by the dieter swallowing the glassful 'I've had my diet, now for my breakfast'.

Rosemary Conley and *Weight Watchers* have weekly meetings with public weighing. *Rosemary Conley* prescribes a low-fat controlled-calorie eating plan and emphasizes exercise. The diet enables most to lose weight without the music-accompanied exercise – a deterrent to some, especially the few men assigned to it. *Weight Watchers* promote a low saturated-fat intake with an allowance of daily 'Points' to avoid complexity of calorie counting. All these three traditional methods use calorie restriction for weight loss. They work if the customer obeys the rules. Many don't, having abandoned responsibility they want to see what rules can be disobeyed without being found out. These three diets are in line with current DoH official advice. The fourth plan, the *Atkins New Diet Revolution*, is not. Nor is it new, but based on Yudkin.

A Victorian undertaker, William Banting (1796-1878). promoted a similar approach in the 19th century As a philanthropist he provided the information free. Atkins is the most controversial, and though over 35 years old, it was in the best-seller lists in the UK for many years, and 10 million books sold in the USA since 1972, despite (or perhaps because of) severe criticism from USA cardiologists and from most nutritionists.

The medical profession has a dismal record here. To oppose Atkins because he advocates high fat intake lacks credibility because 30 years ago the profession recommended a similar regime when it was fashionable to decry carbohydrates.

Those who can afford Atkins recipes are the affluent. After his death (April 2003) his diet became for a time more fashionable in the UK. Not so in most European countries. Would the French give up baguettes, the Italians pasta, the Germans beer, the Spanish rice or all of us potatoes? When physicians disagree, laymen should choose the sensible option. Atkins follows Yudkin and prescribes a cut in carbohydrates so drastic as to induce ketosis. This burns up surplus fat, and also muscle. When the target is achieved the muscle deficit has to be restored so the fat lost is less than the weight loss claimed. Ketosis is a metabolic change, accompanied by halitosis, constipation, nausea and lassitude. It is indefensible to force the healthy into ketosis, so they can go on eating more than they need; nearly everyone can digest carbohydrates normally.

Because the *Atkins Diet* works supporters say it should be used. Any scheme that forbids victims a major component of normal food intake is bound to work. This is equivalent to justifying the use of a tapeworm; it also produces weight loss; the parasite is killed and expelled when no longer needed. Would that be ethically acceptable?

Few medical colleagues can ethically recommend Atkins to patients. Encouraging gluttony (as much fat and protein as one wants), and forbidding carbohydrates are both to be deplored. The fundamental ethical objection is the infliction of ketosis on unsupervised dieters on the false premise that most overweight people, now more than half the population, cannot digest carbohydrates, because they are said to have a metabolic disorder. The evidence for this is flawed (see Letter 8). The commonsense view is they eat more than they need. The only good reason for inducing ketosis to produce weight loss is when treating morbid obesity as a medical emergency, as, for example, when supervised 'compassionate starvation' for a short period was used in Bristol (see Letter 11) to demonstrate to volunteers that everybody can lose weight. Imposing ketosis unsupervised and at random is unacceptable.

Encouraging gluttony is not good advice for the overweight. Nor does it teach restraint, needed when the diet ends. The prescription of low carbohydrate for the rest of one's life with no prospect of ever returning to a normal or even a modest carbohydrate intake is an unpalatable regime, which quickly palls. It was the only diet for which Surrey University felt obliged to test kidney function by a monthly blood sample. Food bills are doubled; adding insult to injury, expensive vitamin and mineral supplements are needed to replace the nutrients lacking because of the low carbohydrate intake. The Atkins foundation makes more profit from supplements bought by the gullible than from sales of their books.

And yet there are still many who recommend the Atkins Diet because 'it works'. So as this plan leaves the decision to you, it is entirely up to you whether, despite the arguments above, you would still contemplate using it as a last resort to lose weight quickly. But remember the warnings and use your commonsense if complications happen.

Viewers of the *Diet Trials* TV programmes hoping for enlightenment were dismayed by the attitude of those on screen – TV performers at their worst, self-indulgent, shallow and jokily articulate. Many viewers were appalled by the lack of restraint and by the willingness of sapient beings to submit to rules at odds with commonsense. An objection to all these diets: having to do what you are told. The failure of all four was an inconclusive but appropriate result.

Letter 20: Is Food Addiction a Problem?

Dear H

Some psychiatrists assert obesity is usually due to food addiction. As they claim expertise in treating addiction, with half the population now overweight, they are claiming jurisdiction over millions. We all need food but it is absurd to say we are addicted to it, because we enjoy it; it is part of normal living. We can be habituated to three meals a day, but that is not addiction. A very small minority, correctly diagnosed as addicted to food, are mentally ill. Theodore Dalrymple's book Junk Medicine is relevant to this subject; see the Appendix.

A fundamental mistake that bedevils most discussion on the vexed question of addiction is concentrating on the addictive item. Puritans believe what we enjoy is bad for us and should be forbidden. The common addictions, to alcohol, nicotine, cannabis, heroin, cocaine and other drugs, are discussed in the context of how to control these substances, and how to prevent them from falling into the hands of a public not trusted to use them sensibly. If food is addictive, it should be in the above list, which is absurd.

It is putting the cart before the horse. The addictive item is not the main problem, though it deserves consideration. The question should be: who are the addicts? The addictive people are the problem. Those addicted to one item, if it is unavailable, transfer their addiction to another. Using an alternative drug to wean addicts from their chosen fix is thus a predictable failure. Addicts misuse drugs, alcohol and tobacco. They are inadequate personalities, with a tendency to obsessive and manipulative behaviour.

The argument is supported when we look at other addictions, to activities rather than substances: computer games, football, gymnastics, cards, gambling, running, jogging. The list is long, and can include eating, in place of food in the previous list. As the evil of addiction is not due to the items abused, the argument about how they should be controlled is irrelevant. Even the most vociferous have not yet recommended restricting food by law to make us healthier though they are getting near. The anti-tobacco lobby, the anti-alcohol lobby and other single-issue fanatics, are keen to stop us from using these, though both are legally available; indeed their widespread use provides revenue upon which the Treasury depends. Forgotten or ignored by those campaigning for abolition is the failure of Prohibition nearly 80 years ago in the USA. Alistair Cooke summarized this recently: 'Been there, done that'.

With cannabis partially derestricted, whether the harder drugs now in common use should be legalised is hotly debated. There seems no recognition that it is not the drugs themselves that cause the problem, but the sad victims who misuse them. Whether they should be protected for their own sake from their own inadequacies raises more questions. At what cost of civil liberty, should further regulations be imposed on the majority? What guarantee is there that any such draconian policy will work? The problem of caring for those enslaved and debased by drugs and the harm to society by criminals intent on stealing to feed a drug habit demands that the policy of eliminating illegal drugs should be made to work. Many see this as unrealistic; the cost of policing, imprisonment of offenders, repair of damage from affrays, all continue with no signs of improvement. The alternative scenario of decriminalising drugs would not help the persistent drug users, though it might remove the financial incentive for mafia-type drug suppliers to continue their sordid occupation.

We are concerned only with the accusation of being addicted to food. We plead innocent. We must be allowed to eat what we want without feeling guilty.

Letter 21: Pessimist and Optimists

Dear H

With regard to weight loss, the lesson insofar as you have a choice, is to be an optimist, not a pessimist. Not only will your odds of success be better. Statistically, you will have a greater chance of good health, and certainly you will be happier.

Optimism and pessimism are relevant to weight control. As a retired GP with long experience of many normal patients, not needing the psychiatric advice that dominates most publications about weight loss, I was fortunate in my practice. The population I served since 1950 were mostly determined to make a success of their lives. They were positive, self-reliant, willing to change occupation when local circumstances demanded, and in general not members of the 'chattering classes'. It was not until the 1960`s when doing sessions for a new deputising service, I saw a different range of patients and realised how fortunate I and my partners were compared with neighbouring colleagues who had to contend with so many pessimists.

Positive people, enthusiastic optimists accept common sense advice. They meet a challenge using their own resources. In contrast negative melancholics, often inadequate personalities, display addictive and manipulative behaviour, have an inbuilt aversion to rational explanation, and need psychiatric help before accepting a new way of life. They demand appetite suppressants, tranquillisers, or sleeping tablets. They resent being told tablets are temporary crutches for an emergency, likely to be habit-forming and ineffective if used long-term. Ultimately they must rely on their own resources. It takes a great deal of time to persuade them; it was tempting to refer them for psychiatric advice, if only so that more time could be given to patients willing to accept advice about changing life-style. The NHS with limited resources since it began, depended for its survival on rationing, either by financial constraints, prescription charges, or time – that is, by appointment systems and waiting lists. It is up to the individual GP to decide how to use the limited time available for the benefit of the majority of his patients. Increased staffing does not produce more time for patients, just as more bureaucracy in hospitals does not mean better services for patients. When the number of administrators exceeds the number of beds, the solution for the inevitable financial crisis is to close wards and sack medical and nursing staff as there is no money to pay them. The possibility of sacking administrative staff is never mentioned. Perhaps this is a jaundiced view from one long retired?

Can we decide individually to become optimists, or is it a matter of our genes? Who knows? Some veer between pessimism and optimism, an extreme example being those with bipolar disorder – it used to be called manic depression. If free will operates here, perhaps some can make a conscious choice.

Letter 22: A Lesson from Venice

Dear H

The intractable progressive obesity problem, recognized as a threat to the whole population, is not going to be solved by the bureaucrats who control NHS policy; they have failed with drugs and addiction to smoking or alcohol. Cannabis as a recreational drug will add to these difficulties, though welcome insofar as it can help those who suffer from the few diseases whose symptoms it can relieve.

One aim of this booklet is to warn that expert opinion is fallible. It is still difficult to persuade many sensible people to start this method of non-drug, non-dietary regime of eating less. Even when convinced this regime works, they still hesitate. Why? Excluding indolence the main reason is fear of being hungry. Irrational – yes – we are all irrational to some extent; the fear of hunger must be met.

On return from a regular visit to Venice, I noticed that some of the local population, especially the young, shows an increasing tendency to being overweight. If you wonder why I should notice this or even how one can tell, with so many tourists there, one answer is that I have become more observant since taking up painting.

We were based on S. Elena, free of tourists. But even in other parts of Venice it is easy to escape them; a few yards off the tourist routes Venetians busily go about their normal affairs, walking purposefully – unlike the wandering tourists.

Venetians, healthier than most Italians, must walk everywhere; even using public transport – water-buses – they often prefer to stand, using their leg and thigh muscles to maintain balance, for example on the non-motorised traghetti crossing the Grand Canal.

They are also fitter because they go up and down the steps to the bridges over the numerous canals crossed on most journeys. Our Venetian grandchildren can out-walk their contemporaries when they come here in the summer. Yet despite living in an environment with the built-in facilities of a gym (the steps to the bridges) and enjoying the reputedly healthy *Mediterranean diet* rich in fish and olive oil, obesity is increasing, even among the young. The arrival of MacDonald's has not helped but the problem began before that with the steady gradual relentless increase in the size of food portions that accompany affluence.

Visiting other European countries teaches the same lesson, but most dramatically it is obvious to visitors to the USA. The supplementary question, how can the epidemic of obesity among the young be reversed, is challenging, but a younger generation should find the answer.

Advice for the new millennium is directed at the psychiatrically challenged; the hope is to change the impulses that cause them to overeat by altering their behaviour with drugs or psychiatric therapy. The aim is to control appetite and metabolic rates with food supplements and drugs. Experts cannot agree how to do this. A recent generation of drugs claims to alter serotonin levels, to stop fat being stored, or to act on the brain to switch off hunger. They fool the brain into believing that hunger has been abolished; they are said to be relatively free of side effects. Tablets prescribable only for severe obesity are given only after the chosen recipient has succeeded in losing a specified amount of weight. If weight loss is possible by dieting, why not persevere with that alone? Using drugs powerful enough to fool the brain are likely to have undesirable actions on other parts of the nervous system. The idea that powerful drugs can cure obesity is inherently dubious. They have no relevance for those committed to non-dietary control of our weight.

Letter 23: Individuality and appetite

Dear H

We forget how singular we all are. We know we have unique fingerprints, DNA, iris recognition patterns, handwriting, writing or painting styles, face features showing remarkable differences, some very subtle. Despite this we are imbued with the idea of fair shares and – a hangover perhaps from the distant days of rationing, or from childhood memories – distributing food equally. But we are all different. We all need differing amounts of food.

We know we cannot quantify our individual needs. We should decide individually what, how and when we should eat. In practice social conventions constrain us. We, who need to moderate our intake because we have a genetic tendency to store fat, must do the best we can individually. With experience we learn our individual needs and how to ignore advice that is wrong for us.

Arguably the most difficult thing to learn is appetite control. A well-known piece of advice: rise from the table before you feel full. It is a common mistake to believe you are still hungry because you don't feel full. Confusion about feeling hungry when merely not replete baffles many. Other tips of this kind are available from books on eating that can be helpful even if the main thesis of a book is not convincing. It is up to each of us to experiment and find our own solution. What works for one may not work for others. Sensations from the abdomen should not be allowed to decide the matter; the decision must be made 'between the ears'. Some find it helps to eat slowly, others find that difficult. Ultimately it is individual self-persuasion, being willing to learn and being prepared to abandon long-held beliefs that will determine whether or not we succeed.

The problem can be considered as a battle between mind and body, the soul and the flesh, perhaps even good and evil. The body tries to conserve reserves; if food fails to come, signals are sent. If ignored more peremptory demands are made. In a culture when all demands of the body have to be met, a snack if not a full meal is considered necessary. The pervasive idea that what is wanted and what is needed are identical, must be confronted and abandoned.

We know it is possible to ignore or at least postpone response to such demands. It can be difficult, but when it comes to a choice, it is for each of us to decide what to do. It is not for others, however well qualified they believe themselves to be, to pontificate. Sources of contradictory advice can be ignored however strident or persuasive.

Finally we must rely on our own resources for symptoms like hunger with a large psychological component. We all have irrational or obsessive impulses, but we know these must be resolved by ourselves using the resources we have, or can summon up to ensure that such impulses are resisted. Each battle won is a good precedent for the future.

It is difficult to write on this subject and escape the trap of encouraging obsession with food so the final letter will suggest possible distractions before a summary of recommendations made in these letters.

Letter 24: Distractions

Dear H

The simplest and most effective method of dealing with the psychological component of hunger, and the consequent craving for food, is distraction.

It is important to discover how to distract ourselves from hunger. We must find something, indeed anything to occupy our thoughts when dominated by food.

You and I know how quickly we can become absorbed in painting or drawing. Those who have experienced this know it is also relaxing and calming though many believe only a minority have a talent to paint or draw. This is not so. Everyone who can use a pen or pencil can learn the basic skills. In the Victorian era every young lady was taught to sketch or paint; most became competent, many proficient and some expert. Sadly it is no longer fashionable. Those who believe they cannot draw should try. Start with *Drawing on the Right Side of the Brain* by Betty Edwards if unwilling to attend a class.

Equally absorbing can be music, ideally participating, though attentive listening can banish thoughts of food. Reading or any hobby can distract us from hunger.

If you have no hobby, enthusiasm is the key to fascination by a new subject; seize any opportunity. Even mathematics can become a special interest, for example: 24 to me is a good round number to complete these letters; if you think 20 – the original number – is a rounder one, it is because we use a decimal system. Two dozen, the number of hours in a day is preferable. A dozen and its multiples up to a gross are widely used in marketing. They are more easily divisible and mathematically more versatile than decimal equivalents. Bach revolutionized music with his 48 preludes and fugues, making equal temperament, a mathematical curiosity itself, practical. Had we been born with 6 digits we would not have started counting in fives or tens. We could have had a duodecimal system with two new names for single integers for ten and eleven, with one/zero representing twelve.

Considering such implications is an example of how to divert the mind from food worries. Proficiency in maths is not needed to appreciate many mathematical puzzles. Hobbies do not require expertise for them to be effective. An amateur painter or musician can get even more pleasure from their subject than many professionals.

Those of us who need to lose weight should appreciate our good fortune in living in an affluent society with such a wide choice of food available. Many resent any suggestion of curbing our intake to anything like that endured by those in less fortunate circumstances. This good fortune implies an obligation, if not a duty, for restraint; we can hope that surplus food could be allocated where it is really needed.

Before listing the dozen points summarizing the message of these letters, and listing a half dozen myths and facts, the final emphasis must be on moderation and restraint; it is of overriding importance that this be given prime consideration in our change of eating habits to ensure that weight lost is not regained. Surveying many schemes, none of which has had any impact on the so-called epidemic of obesity, we come full circle to Letter 1: no need to diet. Eat what we like, though much less of it.

Popular Misconceptions

Myths	Facts
It is impossible for some to lose weight	Obesity vanishes in famine conditions
However little I eat, I remain fat	If you replicate famine conditions, e.g. in a health farm, weight will be shed
I can't resist food	If food is not available, e.g. desert island, exploration, hostage, prison, you will learn the hard way
Hunger demands relief by food	A small amount of food relieves physical hunger. Psychological hunger responds to distraction
My metabolic rate is low so I cannot burn up fat	The active obese often have high metabolic rates, needed to provide the energy expended carrying a burden of weight which the thin would find intolerable
Addicted to food, I cannot stop eating	The addiction is not to food, but to eating. It used to be called gluttony, one of the seven deadly sins, now downgraded to a behavioural disorder. If self-control eludes you, seek spiritual advice for a deadly sin or psychiatric cognitive therapy for the behavioural disorder

For those who start reading a book from the back, here is a summary of the main points

1 Obesity and its precursor, being overweight, affect roughly half of the population.

2 For over fifty years, the proportion of overweight people has increased, as has food consumption, both in step with affluence.

3 The half not affected are genetically fortunate in being able to burn up the excess they eat. This may not last.

4 The half who are affected must make a permanent change in their eating habits.

5 The remedy, for those affected, is to eat less than they think they need.

6 Those affected should accept responsibility; no one else can do it for them.

7 Because we all differ, we must discover our own individual solutions.

8 Counting calories, weighing food, and similar complications are unnecessary; avoid them. Cut down total quantity.

9 Menus, which suit some, will not work for others. Choose your own.

10 Experts offer conflicting and changing advice; ignore them, and any advice that contradicts common sense.

11 Exercise if you want but do not rely on it alone for weight loss. Restricted food intake is vital and is more efficient.

12 Individual responsibility is not practical for children, the irrational, or the dependent. Total intake must be reduced, trial and error being the criterion for each individual, not dogmatic belief in the unsuitability of certain foods.

Appendix: Doubting the Department of Health

"Of all the many values of Science the greatest must be the freedom to doubt"

Richard Feynman, Physicist.

'How to slim' advice for the overweight comes not only from the Department of Health, but also from commercial companies and from the increasing numbers of nutritionists, much of it conflicting. Diets, despite their failure rate of over 90%, are still widely promoted, for example at the well publicized first International Obesity meeting of 200 delegates in South Africa. A pronouncement from Professor Phillip James (Nov 2004), Chair of the International Obesity Task Force – such a body does exist – said: 'The only way we can manage obesity is to get governments involved.' This booklet takes the opposite view. It is for individuals to take back this responsibility. Governments should not be spending taxpayers' money on schemes, which fail in nine cases out of ten, to help those needing to lose weight. It distracts from the real need to reduce food intake.

Surgeons at this conference identified reducing food intake as the main target. Their proposed solution was a peculiarly surgical one — radical keyhole surgery to reduce stomach capacity. This would be an extravagant procedure even for the opulent corpulent. Where what we might call the bulk of the problem is concerned, the obese themselves, it is impossible to take any such suggestion seriously. The numbers involved, the cost, the public outcry at the allocation of resources would rule it out.

Admittedly, every country has its own circumstances. The first conference was in South Africa where USA levels of obesity coexist with large-scale starvation, complicated by the overwhelming presence of HIV infection. Many of the overweight and obese were reluctant to be seen to be losing weight, in case it was attributed to Aids.

None of this should hide the absurdity of a surgical solution to the need to reduce food-intake. It is a forbidding thought that this conference in South Africa was the beginning of a long series of regional meetings, generously sponsored by drug companies scheduled to culminate in a World Obesity Conference three years into the future. Since this happened the experts still ponder. They learn strategies for controlling obesity, but patients do not benefit.

Edicts from the Department of Health pronouncing official policy, including targets set for GPs do not inspire confidence. They come with the stamp of certitude, never a suggestion of possible error. The DoH discourages questioning of its policies, yet certainties have recently been overturned, as in the case of the organism Helicobacter pylori causing peptic ulcer (see Letter 7). The U-turn regarding 'Helicobacter pylori' was not an isolated event. Previous reversals of treatment have been accepted by the DoH, usually ungraciously. We must follow Professor Feynman's advice and we must doubt – even those of us with perhaps a natural reluctance to question advice from Government sources.

Precedents for challenging orthodoxies should be cited if *"Evidence-Based Treatment"* is to be embraced. According to Dr David Eddy, in the USA only 15% of what doctors do is backed by hard evidence. Claiming medicine is an art rather than a science is not a good answer nor will it attract funding when competing with alternative therapies, despite Voltaire's dictum: ***"The art of medicine consists in amusing the patient while nature cures the disease."***

The fundamental fallacy of DoH policy is focusing on treatment of the 'average' – wrongly taken as equivalent to 'normal'. Such an approach fails where individual reactions vary widely. The DoH looks at large numbers, in the attempt to improve health nationwide. A GP, by contrast, sees an individual patient. Treatment for an individual is not the same as that advised for a large group. Dietary advice must be geared to the individual, to accommodate their particular variations.

This disagreement is one cause of the misunderstanding (or frank hostility) that exists between the DoH and many of the doctors it supervises. Another is the cavalier response when DoH advice is questioned. When controversial dietary advice for all is promoted, GPs as independent contractors legitimately have reservations. But the

DoH, having decided policy (through a committee), disregards contrary opinions from GPs.

The status of GPs as independent contractors is ignored. This was the designation when the NHS was inaugurated. I remember cynics at the time believed it was to avoid the Government being responsible for holiday arrangements. When the NHS started in July 1948 I was running, with no bureaucratic restrictions, for the widow of a GP, his single-handed practice of 4,500 patients until the ownership of the practice would be taken over by the NHS. Not many remember the time when practices were bought and sold. This was one of the first to be awarded to a GP applicant.

Now there are 'traffic lights' to label foods that are in or out of favour, targets for blood pressure, cholesterol and salt levels. None of these is open for discussion – it is not even admitted that they might be controversial.

Authority's first tactic is to ignore alternative options. Pretending they do not exist does not make them go away and is foolish when so many have access to the Internet. For the first time patients have unparalleled access to alternative specialist advice to that promulgated by the DoH. Anyone interested, for example, in salt or cholesterol will find that all 'experts' do not share the universal abhorrence with which health advisors and the compliant media regard these. The disputed facts, whether right or wrong, are not the issue. It is the attempt to conceal or deny the existence of alternatives that is deplorable.

The lack of tolerance for minority opinions, the assumption that all problems can be answered by a simple yes or no, raises suspicions. Answers in the categories of 'possible', 'probable', 'unlikely' or 'unknown' are ignored. Mathematicians would consider such options as theories, hypotheses or conjectures. In Mathematics once a proof is accepted, it becomes a theorem: a proposition that has been rigorously proven and is known to be objectively true. Medicine is not yet ready for this – perhaps still too much art, not enough science.

A simple example: Salt

Alleged, but not universally agreed, to be a cause of high blood pressure, salt is vital for sodium balance. Too little and we are in trouble with leg cramps, while common sense tells us too much is fatal – drinking seawater for example. So we need to get the balance (dose) right. Current DoH advice is 6g intake daily maximum. Many conscientious followers of official advice will take far less, so a substantial number will get muscle cramps. Other experts advise 12g as a sensible limit. Japanese take double this without ill effect. Our self-regulating systems are efficient in retaining the salt we need and excreting the surplus in sweat or urine. Is it sensible or ethical to limit everyone's intake in case it harms a few? Eating too much food causes some to take too much salt. **When food portions are reduced to a sensible level there is less need to worry about our salt intake.**

A complex example: Cholesterol

Voltaire (1694-1778): It is dangerous to be right in matters on which the established authorities are wrong.

The case of cholesterol is more controversial. Demonised as a cause of heart attacks, cholesterol is a vital component in our body, being a precursor of important enzymes. Its blood level is the cause of much anxiety, made worse by the assumption that its level in the bloodstream is related to the cholesterol in our diet. Physiologists know this is not true.

Dr Richard Asher (1912-1969) the much admired medical writer and teacher in the late 60's wrote: "Please do not write any more articles about cholesterol and coronary disease and the diet and drugs which are supposed to influence them. The facts about coronary disease are these: the less atheromatous your ancestors, the harder your (tap) water, and the more habitual exercise you take, the less likely you are to be troubled by it. Do stop bothering about whether your fats are saturated or unsaturated, help yourselves liberally to butter and stop propagating these erroneous legends,"

Dr Malcom Kendrick has long argued against the 'cholesterol myth'. The cholesterol in our blood comes not from cholesterol in our diet but from what we each manufacture ourselves.

Cholesterol levels are capricious. According to Professor Vijay Kakkar many of the 2.7 million in South Asia killed annually by cardio-vascular disease have normal or even low cholesterol levels. These do not reliably predict cardio-vascular disease so the DoH's bribing GPs to persuade patients to have these levels measured is indefensible.

Common sense suggests that these blood levels may be of no significance – they differ markedly for each individual. Yet DoH 'experts' are complicit in allowing false information to be used when they promote 'low cholesterol' (green label) foods and warn that 'high cholesterol' (red label) food is bad. Both are completely changed in the stomach, as are high and low density fats. Blood fat levels and blood cholesterol levels are unrelated to what we eat. Expensive cholesterol-lowering drugs have no place in the treatment of obesity.

Cholesterol levels have been obsessively discussed in the USA since Alistair Cooke told the American Heart Association over forty years ago that, even then, 'cholesterol' had acquired the same connotation as the word 'unclean', used in biblical times to herald the approach of a leper. In November 2003, on the same theme, he told us 'every American, from a bishop to a truck driver knows his cholesterol count; every woman, from a cleaning lady to a psychoanalyst, knows hers; all fear their level will go above normal.' In the UK, though encouraged by the DoH to worry, few know their level. In France even fewer bother. The intention was to reduce heart attacks and to cut obesity. The latter has steadily increased.

One cholesterol conference failed even to agree normal levels because of the awkward fact that many with naturally high levels live much longer than expected. Perhaps we all need the gene current in a village in Greece where men with huge cholesterol levels live to be about 100; physicians who describe them as 'walking time bombs' die first!

Supporters of the Atkins Diet claim his high-fat diet does not raise cholesterol levels. This suggests natural levels are less susceptible to influence by diet or drugs than many believe.

Postscript

Common sense takes precedence over scientific arguments in this booklet. It is heartening to know readers of the previous editions recognized this. What has changed since then has been the overwhelming influence of the internet. The general public obtain information from this extraordinary resource but the mainstream media has not understood this. Most people no longer trust the authorities to tell us the truth. This has been demonstrated by the gradual but relentless growth of the bloggers.

For those with access to the Internet, the quantity of information available is daunting. Visiting websites we can be overwhelmed by the sheer volume; it can be difficult to know how much is put there by cranks and whether it is reliable. A simple way to reduce the quantity: when searching via Google, tick the box with the silly title *'I'm feeling lucky'*. Many are reluctant to use this apparent invitation to gamble, but it provides a single result instead of many thousands, very often the one you need. If not, then look at the wider choice.

For example *Numberwatch* includes a perceptive review of Dr James Le Fanu's *The Rise and Fall of Modern Medicine* by Professor John Brignell whose website was primarily concerned with the misuse of numbers and statistics. *Numberwatch* is well written, clear and humorous. Though this is now relatively inactive it provides links to many controversies, for example cholesterol and salt. Professor Brignell, in contrast to 'single issue fanatics,' links those supporting and opposing many issues said by authorities to be already "scientifically decided."

The website of Florida physician (and former Nasa astronaut) Duane Graveline, *spacedoc.net* together with *thincs* (The International Network of Cholesterol Skeptics) both maintain that cholesterol is not the evil substance as described by most of the mainstream medical establishment.

Doubts about the serious side effects of statins are now acknowledged, blunting the campaign to prescribe them to everyone over 50. Patients are more ready to complain, even the medical profession is at last being made aware that the side effects are much more common than when statins were first promoted as the wonder drug of the last century. It is the GPs, rather than the consultants or the deskbound DoH, who are first to hear the complaints.

Meanwhile the medical profession seems more concerned with the harm from climate change and urges us all to campaign for action to reduce carbon emissions. Mainstream science and the media believe that the main reason for climate change is the man-made carbon dioxide content increase in the atmosphere (AGW). The truth may, however, be the other way round. Ice cream consumption increases at warm weather in the summer time, but still the ice cream is not the cause or the reason for the warm weather.

This debate continues, aggravated by the scandals of Climategate. It seems perverse for the medical profession to be concentrating on our abstract theoretical carbon footprint when a more immediate problem is our actual iatrogenic handprint, associated with prescribing powerful drugs to everyone over 50. There are voices in favour of a polypill to be taken by all the population to include protection against high blood pressure, heart failure and even obesity. This will inevitably add to the present incidence of iatrogenic disease. (See Preface if you do not know what iatrogenic means.)

We should embrace two virtues: humility, admitting we cannot change the climate either way, and prudence by reducing iatrogenic disease.

The precedence of common sense is not to decry the relevance of scientific arguments. I welcomed them when *Panic Nation* appeared eighteen months after *Enjoy Eating Less* in January 2004. But common sense is more persuasive when scientific arguments are complicated and difficult for those of us not technically equipped to understand them. But we all (well, nearly all) have common sense, and when scientific arguments are disputed common sense is more persuasive in providing the right answer.

Richard Asher's definition of common sense: '*the capacity to see the obvious even amid confusion, and to do the obviously right thing rather than working to rule, or by dead reckoning*' is apposite. This brings us full circle back to the Preface.

Not a bibliography

This is a list of some books that have helped to keep me up-to-date – much has changed since I studied 'science' at school over 70 years ago; they have also been useful as 'distractions' (*see Letter 24*).

The Rise and Fall of Modern Medicine by James Le Fanu. This and Dr Le Fanu's regular columns in the *Daily Telegraph*, and *Sunday Telegraph* have been an invaluable source of common sense up-to-date knowledge of current practice. His talent to persuade readers that his advice is personal to them and inspire trust is enviable.

Why Us? By Dr James Le Fanu (Harper Press) Another excellent book by James Le Fanu reviewed by AD on Bristol MedChi website.

The Pleasure of Finding Things Out. Professor Richard P. Feynman provides a light-hearted account of the complexities of modern Physics. He emphasizes that scientists must report results that contradict as well as those that support a proposition. His ability to clarify difficult scientific concepts in simple language is akin to that of Dr Richard Asher who has done the same for many medical subjects.

Radar, Hula Hoops, and Playful Pigs, Dr Joe Schwarcz, well known in Canada, describes the fascinating chemistry of everyday life. It is a useful corrective to widespread ignorance of a subject not always well taught.

The Music of the Primes, Professor Marcus du Sautoy describes vividly the lives and the many eccentricities of mathematicians who have wrestled with the problem of prime numbers over the centuries.

A Short History of Nearly Everything, Bill Bryson gives a highly readable overview of much scientific knowledge, discussions and arguments from Archeology to Zoology, and everything between.

Probability 1, Amir Aczel discusses the mathematical implications of probability theory. It provides evidence that common sense intuition can be overturned by mathematical arguments.

Panic Nation, I am grateful to Professor Stanley Feldman, Professor Vincent Marks and the 16 other contributors to the essays: "*Unpicking the Myths we're told about Food and Health.*"

Richard Asher talking sense: *Talking Sense* – an anthology of some of his writings are as relevant now as when they appeared forty or more years ago.

The Great Cholesterol Con by Dr Malcolm Kendrick (John Blake) Reviewed by AD on Bristol Medchi website

Bad Science **by** Ben Goldacre (Harper Perennial) Reviewed by AD on Bristol Medchi website) *see Letter 8*

Junk Medicine by Theodore Dalrymple Reviewed by AD on Bristol Medchi website. *See Letter 20.*

Shadows in Wonderland by Colin Ludlow (Hammersmith Press) 2008 brilliant insights about the current state of the NHS from a patient, with some fascinating comparisons between prisons and hospitals.

The History of Medicine, Money and Politics: Professor Paul Goddard, (Clinical Press) 2008, celebrating the 60th anniversary of the NHS in a critical but balanced manner! A fascinating and searching book for all those involved in health-care, and relevant to those embarking on reform of health-care, (in the USA for example) and how some problems could be avoided.